SHHH SECRET

PART-3

FASTER HAIR GROWTH EASY TIPS REVEALED

GARRIEMA SHAH

Why I Wrote This Book

I wrote this book because everyone wants to look beautiful in each and every aspect of their body. My first nonfiction book was on healthy beautiful skin, "Shhh….Secret" that was the Part-1, then I started getting list of queries on hair problems. After replying to their queries one by one I thought of writing a book on long and strong hair. And this book will serve the purpose of providing tricks on hair to everyone, anyone can read it anywhere, plus it will ease up my work also as I do not have to reply one by one.

Hair is often perceived as an extension of a woman's beauty - so who would not want shiny long locks. Lots of people desire an effective and healthy hair growth. There are many benefits of having long and lustrous hair, one is the more hair styles you can try, and who doesn't like experimenting with different styles? Everyone of us loves to dress up like a diva!

Second it enhances your beauty, third, it is a centre of male's attraction. Fourth, it gives you an edge over others which makes you look unique. However, getting your hair grow long and waiting for your desire to be fulfilled can be a tedious task unless you have the right ingredients at your disposal.

I wanted to make this very clear that practically it is not possible to grow long hair in a week or in a month. It is possible only if someone religiously follows natural hair care guidelines. I have piled up all the necessary home made remedies for longer hair growth. There are some remedies which are easy to make and use but there are also some complicated remedies which will require your time. By complicated it doesn't mean that you have to make mixture all by yourself, no. But some techniques in which you have to boil the mixture, cool down and strain the liquid.

So girls out there looking for some small, simple and easy to use solutions for a faster hair growth can go through the contents of the book and step-by-step try the remedies. Wait for 2 weeks and you will see the difference!

Why You Should Read This Book

This book will help you to gain your knowledge of how to stimulate hair growth instantly. It is quite understandable in this digital generation that you may be flooded with daily blogs, articles, e-books and websites regarding natural and effective longer hair care growth. But what makes this book different from other sources of information is that here in this book, you will get to know about secret remedies which were tried and it gave desired results.

We all know what diet we have to inculcate in our daily routine, therefore I have not mentioned about following diet or healthy foods. You all are smart and educated enough to know what should be included in our daily diet which is beneficial for our natural hair and skin care. So there is no point stating that again and again. You will find only remedies and easy-to use applications for effective hair growth without any side effects.

I am against the philosophy of eating any pill for hair growth specifically! I always believe in kitchen secrets since my childhood and I have applied all the mentioned technique in this book on my hair and experienced an instant result in two and a half weeks of time. It was an inch of my hair length increased in two and a half weeks of time! You wont believe me! But that is the fact. You have to trust me on this part.

"The hair is the richest ornament of women"

<u>Martin Luther</u>

EFFECTIVE WORKABLE SECRETS FOR LONGER HEALTHY HAIR

Hair are the most important part of any female's beauty and every girl wants to be the centre of attraction amongst her peers. No matter what we are, where we belong to, what we do, it hardly matters whether you are a small town girl, metro girl, working lady or housewife. Even small town girls have an added advantage over other females who stay in big metropolitan cities. They are aware of kitchen found beauty secrets and they apply as well, they stay in pollution-free zone so there is a least possibility of getting exposed to dust and this way their skin and hair are protected.

Every girl or women in any part of earth is conscious about her hair. We all have observed, experienced and digested the fact that there are some lot of "lucky girls" who are gifted with long lustrous hair. They do not have to work hard on their hair's growth, they have the natural tendency of rapid hair growth, but there are some girls who feel themselves to be "unlucky" as they are not gifted with long hair. And I was one of those unlucky girls until I found the secret for faster hair growth. There might be several reasons for natural efficient growth of long hairs, but two of the main reasons for quick hair growth is:

• <u>Heredity</u>

• <u>Healthy lifestyle</u>

Most of the girls desire for long lustrous and strong hair. Growing hair sometimes comes with never ending struggles like awkwardly waiting for length to increase, bouts of hair loss and constant frustrated urge to chop it all off. As a result one gets entangled in this vicious circle of finding quicker ways to grow long hair in a short span of time in getting rich quick kind of schemes.

Some expensive products claim and guarantee for long tresses in 4 weeks. What do you think about "long & strong" and "Faster hair growth" labels you see around yourselves? how should a person get to know what is to be put on hair for better growth? Out of curiosity many girls buy expensive products in desire of getting long hair, but in this painful long journey they get frustrated. And the result is waste of money and time. One of the easiest way is to choose the products that are free of harmful chemicals, or the best option is you can make you own cost effective home made products.

As a matter of fact, there are effective home made remedies present in your kitchen to make your hair grow long not in a short span but in a certain period of time. I am not guaranteeing you that a miracle would happen and your hair will grow 4-5 inches in one night, no that is not practically possible, you need to be patient enough to see the desired results in a 4 weeks of time, which could be around 2-3 inches. All I can say is by religiously following the below mentioned steps on a routine basis can offer you good and healthy hair growth. But you need to take out 1 hour of your time every day, then only it can happen.

All you have to do is prepare below mentioned solutions and keep it somewhere or you can make the paste before applying as well. Preparation method will take maximum 4-5 minutes of your time, applying will take another 5 minutes and then you have to sit back and relax for 20-60 minutes depending on which technique you are following.

"Beauty draws us with a single hair"

<u>Alexander Pope</u>

Some of the girls have it in their genes while some religiously follow healthy lifestyle for quick growth of hair. Most of us crave for healthy, dense and long hair and it becomes very depressing when our hair stops growing. Normal person's natural hair growth is minimum of quarter an inch per month, if it seems to grow at a lesser rate, then There might be several reasons for lesser hair growth are listed:

1. Pollution - If your hair are exposed to pollution and dust, then gaseous pollutants, dust and smoke can all settle on both the hair and scalp causing irritation and damage. It can cause dryness to breakage to an itchy scalp. People who live in highly-polluted areas are more prone to risk.

2. Hard chemicals - Complex prolonged chemical treatments such as hair straightening, smoothing, rebounding, curling not only reduces the quality of your hair but they also makes them dull, lifeless, prone to breakage and it can seriously slow down hair growth as well. You need to take precautionary measures to protect your hair from strong chemicals by applying herbal hair mask, regular hair spa in an interval of 15 days.

3. Hair breakage - After reaching a certain length of normal hair growth it starts to break. Colouring, bleaching, showering, brushing and rough handling of hair can leads to hair breakage. Hairs have this tendency to grow half an inch per month, then it breaks off at the same rate, there might be a possibility of little hair growth or no growth at all.

4. Split ends: Some girls try to maintain the length of hair by avoiding haircut but the net result is no further growth. Hair starts splitting from ends after reaching a desired limit creating thinner strands thereby causing breakage. It is very necessary to trim your hair every 10-12 weeks to avoid split ends. DO NOT WORRY ! TRIMMING DOESN'T NECESSARILY MEAN THAT IT WILL SHORTEN YOUR HAIR. YOU HAVE TO MAKE SURE TO YOUR HAIR DRESSER THAT YOU NEED TO TRIM YOUR HAIR OR REMOVE SPLIT RNDS WHICH WILL CAUSE AN INCH OF HAIR.

5. Stylers and blowers- the high temperatures which are used to design trendy hairstyle damage the cuticles of the hair shaft and thus, reduces hair growth. In order to avoid intense damage of your hair, you can use protective serums. To a certain extent it may protect your hair from damage.

"Long hair is considered bohemian, which may be why I grew it, but I keep it long because I love the way it feels, part cloak, part fan, part mane, part security blanket."

<u>Marge Piercy</u>

<u>Disclaimer</u>- The techniques which have worked for me may not entirely work for you, but at the end it is your hair journey. You need to find out from this book what is best for your hair. And I found all these steps quite beneficial and it has acted as a catalyst for my hair, so why not you also give it a try!

GROWING LONG HAIR TECHNIQUES REVEALED!

Initially I would advise to follow simple and easy-to use methods then by time you will become familiar with procedures you can use some complex methods of making remedies for effective hair growth. Someone has truly said, "No Pain, No gains"

Get ready to take some pains of preparing cost-effective treatments for hair. Here are some easy-to use preparatory steps for quicker hair growth -

1. Honey + Egg mask

Eggs are rich in protein and biotin; it contains potassium, magnesium and albumin which provides nourishment, improves hair growth and lustre in your tresses. They also prevent hair breakage by conditioning the scalp and enhances hair growth too. While honey is loaded with magnesium, potassium, iron, phosphorous and copper. It helps in retaining hydration of the hair structure. So the combination of honey and egg mask is appropriate for hair problems.

APPLICATION :

Mix 1 tbsp of honey with 1 egg and beat until smooth. Apply the mask starting from scalp to the ends of your hair. Soak for about 20-25 minutes, wash it off with shampoo to remove foul smell of egg.

2. Aloe Vera + Fenugreek powder

Being a miracle plant is an ideal remedy for solving majority of hair problems. It is one of the ancient plants to provide extra-benefits for skin, health and weight loss. It is a rich source of Vitamin C, E, Beta-carotene and it contains proteolytic enzymes which repairs dead skin cells on the scalp. Aloe Vera gel promotes hair growth, reduces dandruff and conditions your hair. It has a chemical which is of similar to keratin which has the tendency to rejuvenate hair with its own protein nutrients thereby preventing hair from breakage.

APPLICATION :

It is recommended to use aloevera in its natural form by extracting the gel from the leaf. You can also add other natural ingredients like honey and lemon juice to make your hair more soft, shiny and clear. Cut an aloevera and extract the gel with your hands or spoon, add 1-2 tbsp of fenugreek powder(methi). Apply this mixture on your scalp till the hair ends using your fingers. Leave it for 15-20 minutes and then wash off with shampoo.

3. Vitamin E capsules

There are endless number of beauty products which have Vitamin E as the main ingredient. Vitamin E has antioxidant properties which helps to reduce inflammation and repair damaged hair follicles and these healthy follicles promote hair growth. It is a complete nourishment for your hair.

APPLICATION :

Squeeze 10-20 vitamin E capsules, depending on the length of your hair and extract the oil from the capsule. If the oil is thick then mix it with essential oils like coconut oil, best results with Amla oil. Rub the mixture on the scalp gently. After 30 minutes wash off your hair as usual. Do this remedy twice a week for better results.

4.Red chillies(Cayenne pepper)

I know it sounds very strange, even I was also scared when I heard about this red chilly technique. But believe me it is the topmost secret for efficient growth of hair, this is the tried and tested technique by me. It contains alkaloid capsaicin which improves blood circulation and stimulates hair growth. Scary treatment isn't it? If used in right quantity will show amazing results without any side effects. Trying or not trying is a matter of personal choice, however you may skip to other natural remedies for fast hair growth.

APPLICATION :

Mix pinch (depending on your hair and scalp size) of red chilly with water. If you want to dilute it more then you can add honey and aloe Vera gel as well. Honey and Aloevera will help you out in softening and moisturising of your hair. You can keep this paste for 5-10 minutes, then wash off with regular water or if you want you can shampoo it. If you have the capacity to resist the red chilly for some more time then you can keep it for half an hour as well. It depends on person to person.

PLEASE NOTE: If itching occurs in first few minutes then immediately wash off your hair with shampoo and conditioner, try another technique. Or if you have undergone some hair medication treatment, then do not apply this technique. See below for other suitable ones for you.

Now after applying the above mentioned simple procedures for two weeks you are now good to go with the advanced techniques for faster hair growth. Bit of complicated techniques are listed in this chapter wherein you have to boil some of the mixtures and wait for it to cool down. You have to invest more of your time in preparing the remedies. Do not worry below mentioned techniques will not eat up your day, it will just require your concentration and a bit of patience. So be calm and patient while preparing the mixture!

5. Onion juice

Onion have anti-bacterial properties, which improves blood circulation thereby contributing to faster hair growth. It is rich in sulphur(minimise breakage and thinning), being a good anti-oxidant it reverses the effects of premature greying.

APPLICATION :

Extracting juice from onion is a cumbersome task. Peel off onion And grate it on a plate. Rub the small pieces into your scalp in circular movements. Let it sit for half an hour at least or an hour if possible. Then wash off completely. If you have enough time on your week off then you can extract onion juice from 2-3 onions and pour it on your shampoo bottle for more benefits.

PLEASE NOTE: If smell sticks to your scalp after shampooing also then you can avoid going outside for some time. Or you can apply some leave-in conditioner to counteract the foul smell.

6. Amla (commonly known as Indian Gooseberry) powder

Indian gooseberry has been used since ancient times to enhance strength of hair. Massaging Amla on your hair boost blood circulation, which in turn provides nourishment to your follicles and increases hair growth. It is rich in Vitamin C and extremely rich in antioxidants.

APPLICATION :

Pour required amount of amla powder in bowl, add some water into the bowl. Let the powder rests on water for overnight. In the morning apply the paste onto the scalp, leave it for 20-30 minutes, wash it off with plain water.

PLEASE NOTE : DO NOT USE SHAMPOO IMMEDI-
ATELY AFTER THE APPLICATION AS IT MAY BLOCK
AMLA'S MAGICAL QUALITIES OF INCREASING
HAIR.

**You can opt for Amla oil as your regular oil for best ef-
fective results**

7. Henna

It has antimicrobial properties which maintain scalp health,
balances oil production and pH of your scalp. Not only it
will help your hair grow faster, but it also improve hair tex-
ture.

APPLICATION :
Take half cup of henna powder in a bowl, add water to it
and make a thick paste. Set this aside for overnight for the
colour to develop. In the next morning apply paste on scalp
and hair length, wait for 1-2 hours, then wash off with plain
water. Shampoo your hair next day as direct shampooing
after henna will not give desired results immediately. So
shampoo at least after 24 hours.

8. Fenugreek powder

Fenugreek, commonly referred as "Methi" in Hindi, Its leaves are served in India as a vegetable. It contains Protein, which helps fight baldness, it is rich in Potassium, which prevents grey hair. It is a rich source of nicotinic acid, which encourages hair growth. Fenugreek consists of Vitamin A, B, K and C; Potassium, Calcium, Iron and Protein.

APPLICATION :

Mix 2 tablespoons of fenugreek seeds to 1 tablespoon of coconut oil and boil the mixture until the seeds turn reddish. Let the oil cool down and remove the seeds. Massage this oil on your scalp and hair, leave it overnight and wash off next morning. Apply this remedy twice a week for better results.

9. Ginger

It is one of the best ingredients to promote hair growth. This commonly found household spice has been used since centuries in different Ayurvedic treatment for hair. Whether you want to achieve long tresses or simply control hair loss, this natural ingredient is extremely advantageous. Ginger contains vitamins, minerals, antioxidants, magnesium, potassium, some circulatory agents to increase blood flow through the scalp and it is also rich in fatty acids which help prevent the thinning of hair.

APPLICATION :

Mix 2 tablespoons of grated ginger or paste with your regular oil and 1 tbsp of lemon juice. Leave it on for 30-40 minutes and rinse off with your shampoo.

10. Cinnamon powder

Cinnamon (commonly known as "dalchini" in Hindi is a spice used in many cuisines. It contains finer, manganese, calcium and iron. Many people do not know its hidden quality to cure skin, health and hair problems.

Since centuries, cinnamon has been used as a valuable spice for making hair long, strong and beautiful. It stimulates blood circulation in the body which provides nutrition to hair roots and scalp which leads to strong and beautiful hair.

APPLICATION :

Mix equal proportion of cinnamon powder and honey, apply on the scalp, leave it on for 20 minutes and then wash off thoroughly with normal shampoo.

CAUTION - There will be a possibility that you may have an allergic reaction on the scalp which can cause irritation. So it is generally advised to do a patch test before using the cinnamon on your scalp.

11. Inversion method

Put your head upside down, means your hair will be down immediately, in this way circulation of blood will be promoted. This way you are encouraging your hair to be longer and stronger. Just take your head down for about 4 or 5 minutes a day to see the effect after one month.

12. Garlic

Garlic contains elements such as sulphur, copper, vitamin c, selenium and minerals which are beneficial for hair growth. Copper element in garlic promotes hair growth and thickens your hair. Its general application can boost hair growth and regrowth.

APPLICATION :

Take a garlic clove and rub it on your scalp, wait for an hour then massage your scalp with your normal oil, wash your hair with shampoo.

OR

The easiest way is to add garlic to your shampoo then use it on your hair.

PLEASE NOTE : DO NOT USE GARLIC SHAMPOO MORE THAN TWICE A MONTH, OVERUSE CAN DRY YOUR HAIR AND SCALP.

OR

Crush garlic cloves and apply the juices directly on your scalp. Leave it on for few minutes before washing with shampoo and conditioner.

OR

Grate some garlic cloves and mix it with your regular oil. Boil the mixture, let it cool down and strain the liquid. Keep the liquid in a container and you can apply and massage the oil. After an hour, wash off with shampoo and conditioner. You will see the difference instantly, your hair will become smoother than before. Do this remedy twice a week for best results.

13. Green Tea

Green tea originates from the plant known as "Camellia Sinensis", which undergoes minimal processing, leaving it with more antioxidants and nutrients.

It is these antioxidants as well as the presence of caffeine which help stimulate hair follicles and promotes hair growth. Green tea is a rich source of "panthenol" which is normally used in shampoos and conditioners to strengthen the hair. Natural vitamin C in green tea protects your hair and scalp from sun damage.

APPLICATION :

Add 2 cups water to 1 tea bag of green tea. Heat the mixture, strain the liquid, once the liquid cools down, optionally you can add Aloevera gel and a clove(scalp stimulator). Pour the green tea water into your hair and scalp and leave it for 3 to 5 minutes. Rinse off with cool water. You can use this twice a week for better results.

14. Apple Cider Vinegar

Apple Cider Vinegar is an acidic substance and contains good amounts of acetic acid. It helps lower pH and balance hair health. ACV is rich in vitamins C and B and it is loaded with essential enzymes, amino acids, pectin, vitamins, potassium which strengthen hair follicles and adds volume to the hair by reducing split ends.

APPLICATION :

Add a cup of water to 2-4 tablespoons of vinegar to make your rinse. After you have thoroughly shampooed your hair, pour the mixture over your entire scalp till the length of your hair(be careful not to get into your eyes). Massage the mixture into your scalp, it will stimulate circulation thereby promoting hair growth. After the hair dries, vinegar smell will disappear. After 2 minutes rise out the vinegar. Repeat the process once a week which is recommended for most hair and scalp issues.

15. Castor Oil

Castor oil's extraordinary qualities is it contains anti fungal, anti-inflammatory and antibacterial properties. The inflammation around the hair follicle hinders growth and can result in weaker strands of hair. It also contains various vitamins and minerals which help to boost hair growth.

APPLICATION:

Castor oil has a thick consistency, so you can mix it with coconut oil, olive oil or jojoba oil. Hot the mixture of oils and leave it for sometime to cool down, afterwards, you can apply on the scalp and massage as usual. Rinse off your hair next morning. Maybe you have to rinse twice as castor oil is very thick but afterwards you will see the difference.

These were my 15 tips and tricks for longer hair. However when you search over all the internet you will find n number of ways to grow your hair long. These were tried and tested tips by me and I have personally seen the results but I have waited for a week to see the difference in length. The natural remedies to quickly grow hair in a short period of time is not a miracle but it is a daily hard work which you need to put in everyday then only you will be able to get the maximum benefits out of it. The best thing about trying home remedies is that it does not have any side-effects. It is not just applying one of the above mentioned methods in a day and waiting for instant results to happen, then you won't get anything out of it and you will blame your destiny for short hairs. But rather you have to consistently keep on working on your hair by trying home remedies and one day you will get the positive results.

My other part of this Secret series would be on ***how to naturally straighten your hair at home without any harsh chemical products?***

Yes that is correct, it is possible to naturally straighten your hair using homemade products. Because I know how painful this process of straightening at salon is! Painful because you have to spend lots of money on smoothening, straightening or keratin straightening. And on top of it after few months of this chemical treatment, hair fall starts, hair strand gets weaken and your salon dresser would advise you to continue with your costly shampoos and conditioners related to your type of straightening. You have to visit salon for regular hair spas in order to maintain your healthy hair. At home you can easily straighten your hair with more comfort without any side effects. And the result is guaranteed for sure depending on your hair type.

Wish you all the best for your beauty journey and thanks for reading Secret.

"For me, hair is an accoutrement. Hair is jewellery. It's an accessory"

<u>Jill Scott</u>

If you want to get more information on tricks for long hair, then you can connect with me on:

www.buzzobia.com

About The Author

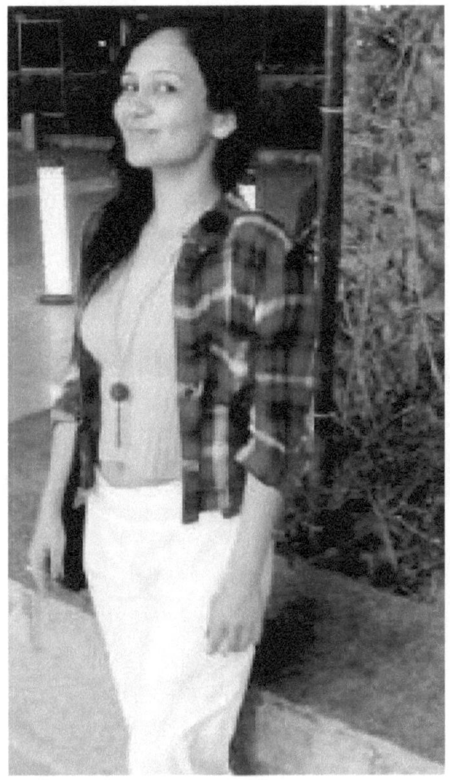

GARRIEMA SHAH is the Amazon author of 2 fiction books -Love is you, U love me? *and 1 non-fiction how-to guide on skin problems - Shhh Secret!.* She lives in Mumbai, India. Garriema loves educating, inspiring and sharing her knowledge and observation with others and live the life of their dreams.

Learn more about Garriema at:

https://authorcentral.amazon.com/gp/profile

OTHER BOOKS BY GARRIEMA SHAH

1. U LOVE ME?

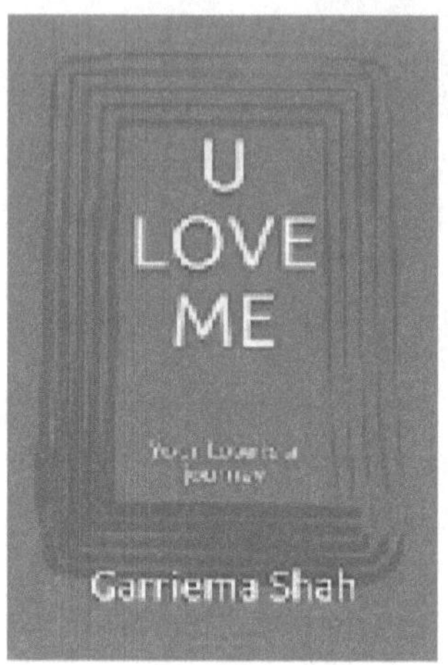

2. Love is You

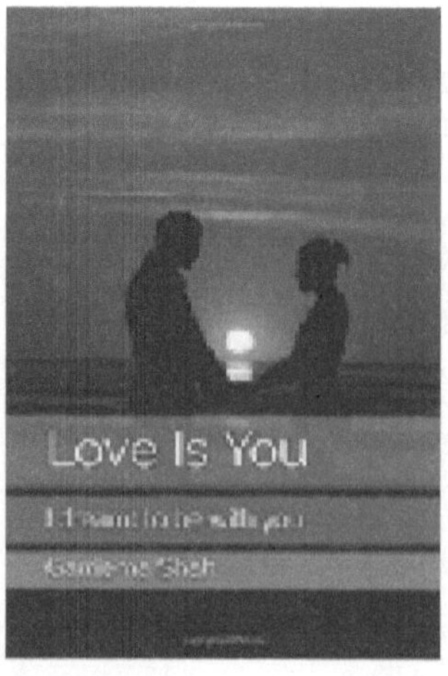

3. Shhhh Secret! - Solution to all beauty problems

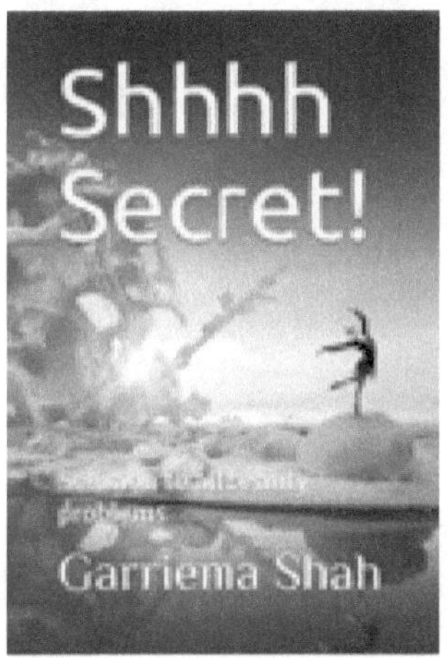

One Last Thing...

If you enjoyed this book or found it useful I'd be very grateful if you'd post a short review on Amazon. Your support really does make a difference and I read all the reviews personally so I can get your feedback and make this book even better.

Thanks again for your support!

www.ingramcontent.com/pod-product-compliance
Lightning Source LLC
Chambersburg PA
CBHW021150260726
48656CB00025B/2330